Ketogenic Air Fryer Cookbook:

Quick and Easy Ketogenic Diet Friendly Air Fryer Recipes for Weight Loss and Healthy Living

Written by

Evelyn Halliday

Contents

Introduction

Welcome to and thank you for choosing **Ketogenic Air Fryer Cookbook: Quick and Easy Ketogenic Diet Friendly Air Fryer Recipes for Weight Loss and Healthy Living.**

The Ketogenic Diet is a phenomenon which has been steadily growing in popularity for almost a decade. It is high in fat, sufficient protein, and low carbohydrate diet designed to aid weight loss, fast, and in the healthiest way possible whilst keeping in great physical shape. Due to its overwhelming results, the Ketogenic diet has taken the world by storm. This low carb diet forces the body to rely on energy in the form of Ketones that are produced by the liver and limiting the amount of energy taken from carbohydrates. This pushes the body into a state called Ketosis which is the body's natural reaction to starvation. The body then uses its stored fats for energy as there are not enough carbohydrates in the system to produce sufficient glucose for energy. A high fat diet helps to counteract the effects of starvation by providing plenty of ketones the body quickly adapts to a life with limited carbohydrates and will begin to look to ketones for its primary source of energy. A properly regulated Ketogenic diet and optimal ketone levels come with many health benefits, including:

- Higher levels of concentration and focus.
- Healthy weight loss.
- Significantly lower blood sugar levels.

- Lower cholesterol.
- Lower blood pressure.
- Improved skin.
- Lower insulin levels.

The Ketogenic diet can sometimes be tricky to stick to especially when attempting to stick to macros as strict as 25g carbs per day whilst still maintaining a calorie intake of 1800-2000 with approximately 175g fats and 100g protein per day. The Recipes in this book aim to support a daily intake similar to the examples above. It is not to be used a strict meal plan as but rather as a supportive guide to help fill in on the days when inspiration is lacking or desire you a change or something a little more exciting and less bland than your regular Ketogenic meal.

Air Fryers are not only the perfect kitchen gadget for Ketogenic dieters they are also fast becoming the 'must have' kitchen gadget and it's easy to see why. Air fired food is incredibly fast and simple to prepare, is fantastically delicious and uses a tiny percentage of cooking oil when compared to regular fryers. This results in much healthier meals with less mess! This book is packed full of delicious Ketogenic diet friendly air fryer recipes but it may also be used as a 'time and temp' directory for those who wish to step beyond the boundaries of the Ketogenic diet.

The 66 recipes within this book were designed to provide and support a number of health benefits, including the normalising of blood pressure and the stabilising and reducing of cholesterol. One of the potential drawbacks to the Ketogenic Diet is increased feelings hunger. When creating the meals for the book this one something that was always kept in the forefront throughout the creative process resulting in recipes that endeavour to provide feelings of fullness that last for longer, leaving the body fully satiated. Diet or not, it is never a good idea to let yourself become weak. All the recipes below have been tried and tested in the real world to prove their suitability in the areas of ease of preparation, flavour, and their compliance in accordance with the fundamentals of the Ketogenic diet. The result is a fantastically varied and delicious selection of only the best of the best Ketogenic friendly meals. The book is divided into sections with recipes suitable for breakfast, lunch, and dinner with a further chapter containing quick to make, tasty snacks and treats that are line with Ketogenic dietary requirements and suited to American cuisine.

Become a healthier happier person today!

Breakfast

The ideal Ketogenic breakfast will leave you satiated, boost your metabolism and help to burn calories. This isn't always easy and that's why below you'll find delicious recipes that take no time at all to prepare. Starting the day with a meal that will protect and guard against inflammation is essential for a number of reasons, one of the main reasons being that inflammation has a huge impact on the body's insulin levels and its sensitivity to it. Cognitive and other degenerative diseases are also impacted by inflammation and weight loss is greatly slowed down or even reversed in those who suffer burst of inflammation. A Ketogenic breakfast works to reduce inflammation within the body by reducing the levels of toxins that build up over time in the bodily system.

Starting the day with a Ketogenic breakfast is not only the ideal accompaniment to any weight loss regime. It will also promote and support healthy blood pressure and blood sugar levels as well as helping the body to purge any allergens and excess fats. When we force our bodies into Ketosis, we are forcing the body to utilise our stored fat reserves and the entirety of the fats and proteins that we consume. This makes eggs the go-to for most Keto breakfasters. They really are the perfect Keto breakfast as they are full of protein and fit effortlessly into the Ketogenic diet, but as with so many ingredients that are good for us, they soon become boring and even tedious. Within the Breakfast chapter of this book, I have endeavoured to make eggs interesting again. However, the recipes below are not overly egg centred, the recipes in this section focus primarily on meats such as bacon, gammon, and steak as the main sources of protein, and I for one LOVE a bacon breakfast. So, let's get stuck in.

Egg and Bacon Breakfast Bakes

Ingredients

6 Large Eggs

4 Slices of Bacon

½ Cup Cheddar or Cashew Cheese, grated

Salt and Ground Pepper to taste

2 tsp of Olive Oil

Method

1. Pre-heat your air-fryer to 380°f.
2. Toss the bacon into the air fryer and cook for 6 minutes.
3. Remove the bacon from the air fryer and chop into small pieces.
4. Drain any excess grease from the air fryer.
5. Coat the insides of 4 ramekins (small oven dishes) with the olive oil.
6. Divide the diced bacon between the 4 ramekins and crack 1 egg into each. Add some salt and ground pepper to taste and 1 teaspoon of milk to each.

Cooking your Egg and Bacon Bakes

1. Pre-heat the air fryer to 380°f

2. Cook for 15 minutes and sprinkle a little cheese on top of each ramekin. Cook for a further 5 minutes or until the egg white sets.

Serving

Serve immediately.

Simple Hard-Boiled Eggs

Ingredients

2-4 Medium or Large Eggs (2 per serving)

Cooking your Simple Hard-Boiled Eggs

1. Pre-heat your air fryer to 340°f.
2. Carefully place the eggs in the air fryer basket and cook for 7 minutes.

Serving

Gently put the Eggs in cold water and allow to cool, this makes peeling them much easier.

Gammon and Pineapple

Ingredients

Gammon Steaks

Pineapple rings, 1 per Gammon Steak

Salt and Ground Pepper to taste

¼ tsp Cayenne Pepper

Method

1. Season the gammon with a little salt and ground black pepper to taste.

Cooking your Air Fried Gammon and Pineapple

1. Pre-heat your air fryer to 380°f.
2. Air fry the gammon steaks for 10-12 minutes or until golden brown, turning midway.

Serving

Top with a pineapple ring, serve hot, with salad (optional).

Bacon and Egg Breakfast Burger

Ingredients

1 Avocado

2 rashers of Bacon

1 medium size Egg

1 large Lettuce leaf

2-5 Spinach leaves

A Thick slice of Tomato

Salt and Ground Black Pepper

Method

1. Carefully cut the avocado in half width-wise (horizontally).
2. Remove the stone and fill the hole with spinach leaves.
3. When the bacon and egg are cooked layer them along with the lettuce and tomato slice on top of one of the avocado halves. Top with the other avocado half.

Cooking your Bacon and Egg Breakfast Burger

1. Pre-heat the air fryer to 380°f.
2. Air fry the steak for 5-7 minutes or a little longer for those who enjoy their bacon extra crispy.

3. Remove the bacon from the air fryer and crack the egg into the air fryer pan still containing the fat from the bacon and cook for 3-5 minutes or until edges begin to brown but the yolk is still runny.

Serving

Enjoy immediately.

BLT Salad

Ingredients

3 Rashers of Bacon

2 Eggs

½ Cup of Spinach

½ Cup of Kale (stems removed)

½ Cup Cherry Tomatoes

½ Cup of Lettuce

1tbl Red Wine Vinegar

Salt and Ground Black Pepper

Cooking your Bacon and Eggs (BLT Salad)

1. Pre-heat your air fryer to 340°f.
2. Carefully place the eggs in the air fryer basket and cook for 7 minutes.
3. Pre-heat the air fryer to 380°f
4. Place the bacon onto the air fryer basket and cook for 4-6 minutes.

Method

1. Chop the bacon rashers.
2. Remove the shells from the eggs and slice.
3. Halve the tomatoes.

4. Mix the spinach, lettuce, kale, and tomatoes in a bowl with the red wine vinegar and a little salt and pepper to taste.
5. Add the bacon and eggs to the mix.

Serving

Serve immediately.

Steak and Eggs

Ingredients

4-6 oz. Sirloin Steak

2 Eggs

¼ Avocado

Salt and Ground Black Pepper

Olive Oil

Method

1. Slice the Avocado and put it to one side.
2. Lightly spray the steak with olive oil and season with salt and ground black pepper to taste.

Cooking your Steak and Eggs

1. Pre-heat your air fryer to 380°f.
2. Place the steak onto the air fryer tray and cook for 4 minutes.
3. Add the eggs to the air fryer, carefully crack the eggs into the air fryer tray next to the steak and cook for a further 8 minutes.

Serving

Slice the steak into bite-size slices and serve alongside the eggs and sliced avocado.

Cloud Eggs

Ingredients

3 Eggs

Salt and Ground Black Pepper

Olive Oil

Method

1. Crack open the eggs and separate the yolks from the whites and place them in different bowls.
2. Whisk the egg whites for 1 minute or until fluffy.
3. Lightly spray the air fryer tray with oil and spoon the whisked egg whites into 3 equal mounds onto the tray.
4. Gently flatten the mounds to about 3cm thickness.
5. Create an impression around 1 cm deep in the centre of each mound of egg whites.
6. Carefully place an egg yolk in the centre of each of the egg white mounds.
7. Lightly season with salt and ground black pepper.

Cooking your Cloud Eggs

1. Pre-heat your air fryer to 380°f.
2. Place the cooking tray onto the air fryer and cook the eggs for 10-12 minutes or until the

whites become golden brown and crispy but the yolk is still slightly runny.

Serving

Serve immediately.

Cauliflower and Bacon Hash

Ingredients

6 Slices of Bacon, roughly chopped

1 Cup of Cauliflower, roughly chopped

½ White Onion, chopped

1 Clove of Garlic, grated

1 tsp Paprika

Slat and Ground Black Pepper

1tbl Fresh Lemon Juice

1 tsp Fresh Parsley, chopped

Olive Oil

Cooking your Bacon

1. Pre-heat the air fryer to 380°f.
2. Place the bacon onto the air fryer basket and cook for 4-6 minutes.

Method

1. Remove the bacon from the air fryer basket.
2. Add the cauliflower, bacon, onion, garlic, paprika, lemon juice to a mixing bowl and add little salt and pepper to taste.
3. Leave to rest for 5-10 minutes.
4. Lightly spray with olive oil before cooking.

Cooking you Cauliflower and Bacon Hash

1. Pre-heat the air fryer to 380°f.
2. Toss the mix into the air fryer basket and cook for 6-8 minutes or until the cauliflower turns golden.

Serving

Serve immediately.

Zucchini Eggs

Ingredients

2 Cups Zucchini

2 Eggs

Salt and Ground Black Pepper

Olive Oil

Method

1. Roughly chop the zucchini into cubes and lightly season with a little salt and pepper to taste.
2. Lightly spray with olive oil before cooking.

Cooking your Zucchini Eggs

1. Pre-heat your air fryer to 360°f.
2. Toss the zucchini into the air fryer tray and cook for 2 minutes.
3. After 2 minutes, crack the eggs on top of the chopped zucchini, wait a few seconds then stir well.
4. Cook for a further 3-4 minutes.

Serving

Serve immediately.

Lunch

By now, we've pretty much burnt off the fats and protein from breakfast. It is important that a Ketogenic lunch has enough fats and protein to get us through to the evening without leaving us feeling drained and weak. Many of the recipes in this section have been designed to be able to be mixed/matched as mains and sides in order to ensure that you are getting as full and varied a diet as possible whilst being able to stick to the guidelines of your own Ketogenic diet plan. There are many different reasons as to why people choose the Ketogenic diet. Many individuals take up the Ketogenic diet in order to combat or reduce symptoms and illnesses. Lunchtime is when we should load ourselves with fats but also, we need to find room for some vegetables (no or low-carb) and a sizable protein boost. The lunchtime recipes below have been chosen due to their practicality and cooking time. Most of us do not have more than 15-20 to spare at lunch and that has been taken into account here. Fast, healthy, delicious is the aim here.

Air Fried Scotch Eggs

Ingredients

400g Ground Pork

5 Eggs

4 Bacon slices

½ tsp Salt

¼ tsp Ground Black Pepper

¼ tsp Paprika

¼ tsp Turmeric

1 tsp Italian Mixed Herbs

½ tsp powdered Garlic

Method

1. Sperate the ground pork in a large mixing bowl, then mix in the salt, ground black pepper, paprika, turmeric, Italian mixed herbs, and garlic and thoroughly mix until fully combined.
2. Place the seasoned ground pork mix in the fridge.
3. Lightly beat one of the eggs and place it in the fridge.

Cooking your Bacon

1. Pre-heat your air fryer to 380°f
2. Toss the bacon into the air fryer basket and cook for 8 minutes or until the bacon begins to crisp.
3. Once cooked chop the bacon into small pieces, as small as you can cut. Then put the bacon to one side.

Cooking your Hard-Boiled Eggs

1. Pre-heat your air fryer to 340°f.
2. Carefully place the eggs in the air fryer basket and cook for 7 minutes.
3. Once cooked, remove the eggs from the air fryer and remove the shells. Then put them to one side

Method

Remove the seasoned ground pork mix from the fridge and separate into 4 equal parts and shape the parts into balls.

1. Take one egg per ball of ground pork and pushing the egg into the centre of the seasoned ground pork, use your hands to shape the ground pork around the egg. Ensure that each egg is thoroughly and evenly covered in the ground pork mix.

2. Remove the beaten egg mix from the fridge and roll each of the covered eggs in the beaten egg mix before rolling them in the chopped bacon pieces.
3. Place in the fridge for 10 minutes.
4. Lightly spray with olive oil before cooking.

Cooking your Air Fried Scotch Eggs

1. Pre-heat your air fryer to 380°f
2. Place the scotch eggs in the air fryer basket and cook for 10-12 minutes or until the scotch eggs turn golden brown.

Serving

Delicious both hot or cold.

Jalapeno Poppers

Ingredients

10-12 Jalapenos, halved vertically

3 Slices of Bacon

7 tbl Cream Cheese

½ Cup Cheddar Cheese, grated

Method

1. Cook and chop the bacon slices as per the cooking instructions below.
2. Microwave the cream cheese for 10 seconds to soften it.
3. Mix together the cream cheese, grated cheddar and bacon pieces in a large bowl.
4. Evenly separate the cheese and bacon mix between the jalapenos.
5. Lightly spray with olive oil before cooking.

Cooking your Jalapeno Poppers

1. Pre-heat your air fryer to 380°f.
2. Place the bacon slices into the air fryer basket and cook for 6 minutes.
3. Finely chop the bacon. (See method above).
4. Set the air fryer to 370°f.

5. Place the jalapeno poppers into the air fryer and
    cook for 5 minutes.

Serving

Serve hot.

Spicy Buffalo Wings

Ingredients

2 Pounds of Chicken Wings

1 Cup of Hot Sauce (see below)

Salt and Ground Black Pepper for seasoning

Ingredients (Hot Sauce)

2tbl of Olive Oil

1 Cup of finely chopped Onion

2 Medium heat Chili Peppers finely chopped

3 Habanero Chili Peppers halved, seeded and finely chopped

3 Cloves of Garlic finely chopped

3 Cups Diced Tomatoes

½ Cup Distilled White Vinegar

2tsp Salt

2tsp of Sugar

Method

Start by making Hot Sauce

1. Heat the olive oil in a saucepan over a medium-high heat. Add the onions, garlic, chili peppers and habaneros to suit your taste. Cook for 4 minutes or until the Onions start to brown, stirring throughout.
2. Lower the hob to medium heat and add the tomatoes, vinegar, salt, pepper, and sugar to suit your taste. Cook for 4 minutes until the tomatoes break down, stir throughout.
3. Pour the sauce from the hob to a blender and puree until smooth.
4. Pour the blended sauce through a sieve and into a bowl and leave to cool.

Preparing your Buffalo Wings

1. Ready the chicken wings by separating the wingtips.
2. Separate the drumettes and winglets and place in a bowl add salt and pepper for seasoning.
3. Evenly cover the chicken with the hot sauce and stir, ensure the chicken is properly coated-marinade for a minimum of 3 hours.

Cooking your Buffalo Wings

1. Pre-heat the air fryer to 400°f.
2. Air fry the chicken for 15 minutes, shake midway.

Serving

Pour the remaining hot sauce over the wings and serve.

Jerk Chicken Wings

Ingredients

2 Pounds of Chicken Wings

½ tsp Cayenne Pepper

1 tsp Paprika

1 tsp Garlic powder

1 tsp Allspice

½ tsp Dried Ginger

¼ tsp Nutmeg

¼ tsp Cinnamon

½ tsp Salt

½ tsp ground black pepper

Method

1. Combine the cayenne pepper, paprika, garlic powder, allspice, dried ginger, nutmeg, cinnamon, salt and ground black pepper in a ziplock or sandwich bag.
2. Ready the chicken wings by separating the wingtips.

3. Separate the drumettes and winglets and place
    in a bowl add salt and pepper for seasoning.
4. Add the chicken to the bag with the Jerk
    marinade and shake, ensure the chicken is
    properly coated- marinade for a minimum of 3
    hours.

Cooking your Jerk Wings

1. Pre-heat the air fryer to 400°f.
2. Air fry the chicken wings for 15 minutes,
    turning midway.

Serving

Pour the remaining Jerk marinade over the wings and
serve.

Ham and Cheese Puff Pastry Parcels

Ingredients

200g Ready-made Puff Pastry

Egg Wash (1 beaten egg with a little milk mixed in)

Mild Cheddar Cheese, grated

1 packed of Ham finely chopped

Method

1. Mix together the chopped ham and grated cheddar in a bowl.
2. Cut the puff pastry into squares between 4cm and 6cm.
3. Place some of the mix in the middle of the pastry squares
4. Moisten the edges of the pastry with egg wash and fold in half into a triangle.
5. Pinch the edges of your pastry triangle to ensure it is properly stuck closed.

Cooking your Ham Cheese Puff Pastry Parcels

1. Pre-heat your air fryer to 390°f.
2. Cook for 10 minutes checking and tossing regularly. Cook up to 8 Ham and Cheese Puff Pastry Parcels per batch.

Serving

Delicious either hot or cold.

Chicken Satay Skewers

Ingredients

500g Chicken Breast, cubed

5tbl Tomato Puree

4 Cloves of Garlic, finely chopped

¼ Onion finely chopped

1tsp Cumin

1tsp Ground Black Pepper

1tbl Sesame Oil

1table Peanut Oil

1tbl Soy Sauce

1tbl Sugar

2tbl Peanut Butter

Half a Lemon

Skewers

Method

1. Put the chicken to one side and combine all the remaining ingredients together in a large mixing bowl.
2. Coat the chicken pieces in the marinade and leave for a minimum of 2 hours to overnight.
3. Before cooking, skewer the chicken pieces approximately 4 pieces per skewer.

Cooking your Chicken Satay Skewers

1. Pre-heat your air fryer to 390°f.
2. Line the basket with foil and place the chicken skewers inside.
3. Cook for 15 minutes turning midway to ensure the chicken is evenly cooked.

Serving

Serve with Rice and a slice of Lime.

Mini Roasted Duck Pies

Ingredients

350g Roasted Duck shredded and finely chopped

½ Red Onion very finely chopped

2tbl Hoisin Sauce

Salt and Ground Black Pepper to taste

Olive Oil

Gow Gee Wrappings

Garnish

Spring Onions thinly sliced

Cucumber Slices

Plum Sauce

Method

1. Mix the chopped/shredded duck with the onion and hoisin sauce, add salt and ground black pepper to taste.
2. Encase some of the mix between 2 gow gee wrappings.
3. Repeat the process for the remainder of the duck, chopped onion and hoisin mix.

4. Lightly spray your mini roasted duck pies with
    olive.

Cooking your Mini Roasted Duck Pies

1. Pre-heat your air fryer to 380°f.
2. Air fry your mini Roasted Duck Pies in batches,
    be sure not to overload your air fryer.
3. Air fry your mini Roasted Duck Pies for 12-14
    minutes turning midway.

Serving

Serve hot with Plum Sauce, Cucumber slices and Spring
Onion garnish or store for later. Delicious both hot or
cold.

Apple and Pork Burgers

Ingredients

350-400g Ground Pork (4 burgers)

1 Avocado per burger

1 ½ Cups of Spinach

2 Apples

Salt and Ground Black Pepper

4 Large slices of Lettuce

2tbl Sesame seeds

Olive Oil

Method

1. Peel and grate the apples, drain off any excess juice and put to one side.
2. Carefully cut the avocado in half width-wise (horizontally).
3. Remove the stone and fill the hole with spinach leaves.
4. Separate the ground pork in a mixing bowl and add the grated apples along with a little salt and pepper to taste.

5. Using your hands combine the ground pork with the grated apple. Ensure the ingredients are evenly mixed.
6. Once fully combines use your hands to form 4 equal sized burger shapes from the mix. The burgers should be around 2cm thick.

Cooking your Apple and Pork Burgers

1. Pre-heat your air fryer to 380°f.
2. Lightly spray the burgers with olive oil before cooking'
3. Place the burgers into the air fryer basket and cook for 14-15 minutes, turning midway.

Serving

When the burgers are cooked layer them along with the lettuce on top of one of the avocado halves. Top with the other avocado half and sprinkle with a few sesame seeds.

Bacon and Broccoli Hash

Ingredients

6 Slices of Bacon, roughly chopped

2 cups of chopped Broccoli

1 cup of Brussel Sprouts, cut into halves

½ White Onion

1 Clove of Garlic, grated

Olive Oil

Salt and Ground Black Pepper

Method

1. Mix all of the ingredients together in a mixing bowl.
2. Season the mix with salt and ground black pepper to taste.
3. Lightly spray with olive oil before cooking.

Cooking your Bacon and Broccoli Hash

1. Pre-heat your air fryer to 380°f.
2. Toss the mix into the air fryer basket and cook for 8-10 minutes.

3. Remove the air fryer basket and its contents
    from the air fryer and place the air fryer tray
    into the air fryer to warm up.
4. Lightly spray the air fryer tray with olive oil and
    crack the egg onto the air fryer tray and cook or
    5-6 minutes.

Serving

Place the fried egg on top of the bacon and broccoli
hash and enjoy.

Bacon wrapped Asparagus and Avocado Fries

Ingredients

1 Pack of Asparagus

1 Avocado

1 Slice of Bacon per Asparagus Stalk/Avocado slice

Method

1. Slice the Avocado in half and remove the stone.
2. cut each avocado half into 5 equal slices and carefully remove the skins.
3. Carefully wrap each avocado slice and asparagus stalk with a slice of bacon.
4. Lightly spray with olive oil before cooking.

Cooking your Bacon Wrapped Asparagus

1. Pre-heat your air fryer to 380°f.
2. Toss the bacon wrapped avocado and asparagus into the air fryer basket and cook for 12-14 minutes or until the bacon is golden and beginning to crisp.

Serving

Serve immediately.

Cauliflower Fritters

Ingredients

1 Cauliflower

2 Eggs

½ Cup Almond Flour

½ tsp Turmeric

½ tsp Paprika

Salt and Ground Black Pepper

Olive Oil

1 Pan of Water

Method

1. Break the cauliflower into florets and add to a pan of boiling water for 8 minutes.
2. Remove the cauliflower from the boiling water and toss into a food processor or blender and pulse for 20-30 seconds.
3. Toss the cauliflower into a mixing bowl and add the almond flour, turmeric, paprika, and a little salt and ground black pepper to taste. Mix well.
4. Using either your hands or a large wooden spoon, form patties from the cauliflower mix.
5. Lightly spray with olive oil before cooking.

Cooking you Cauliflower Fritters

1. Pre-heat your air fryer to 360°f.
2. Gently place the cauliflower fritters into the air fryer basket and cook for 5-7 minutes or until the cauliflower fritters are golden and beginning to crisp.

Serving

Delicious either hot or cold.

Broccoli and Parmesan Fritters

Ingredients

2 Cups chopped Broccoli florets

½ Cup Almond Flour

2 Eggs, lightly beaten

1/2 Cup Parmesan

1 Clove of Garlic, finely chopped

½ tsp Chili Flakes

¼ tsp Salt

½ tsp Ground Black Pepper

Method

1. Boil or steam the broccoli for 5 minutes before draining and allowing to cool. Lightly mash.
2. Mix the almond flour, parmesan, garlic, chili flakes, salt, ground black pepper, and egg. Add the broccoli and combine the mix.
3. Use your hands to form patties from the broccoli and parmesan mix.
4. Lightly spray your fritters with olive oil before cooking.

Cooking your Broccoli and Parmesan Fritters

1. Pre-heat your air fryer to 380°f.
2. Place the broccoli and parmesan fritters in the air fryer basket and cook for 6 minutes or until crisp, turning midway.

Serving

Serve hot with a squeeze of lemon.

Mediterranean Broccoli Salad

Ingredients

2 Cups Broccoli

½ Cup Sun-Dried Tomatoes

¼ Cup Red Onion, finely chopped

¼ Cup Olives, pitted and halved

2 Cloves of Garlic, grated

1 tsp Italian Mixed Herbs

Salt and Ground Black Pepper

Olive oil

½ Cup Greek Yoghurt

1 tbl Fresh Lemon Juice

Method

1. Using a large bowl, mix the broccoli, red onion, sun-dried tomatoes, garlic, olives, Italian mixed herbs.
2. Lightly spray the mix with olive oil and stir thoroughly.

3. In a separate bowl, mix together the Greek yoghurt and fresh lemon juice and leave to one side.

Cooking your Mediterranean broccoli

1. Pre-heat your air fryer to 360°f.
2. Toss the broccoli mix into the air fryer basket and cook for 6-8 minutes.

Serving

Serve with a dollop of the Greek yoghurt and lemon juice mix. Delicious both hot and cold.

Air Fried Thai Haddock

Ingredients

4 Haddock Fillets

1 Inch piece of Ginger, grated

1 Clove of Garlic, grated

2 Lemongrass stalks, finely chopped

1 White Onion, finely chopped

2 Red Chillies seeded and finely chopped

1 tsp Coriander

1 tsp Crushed Peppercorns

2 Kaffir Lime Leaves chopped

1 tbl Sesame Oil

Salt and Ground Black Pepper

Method

1. Combine the ginger, garlic, lemongrass, onion, chillies, coriander, peppercorns, lime leaves, sesame oil, and a little salt and ground black pepper to taste.

2. Completely submerge the haddock in the marinade, fully cover and leave to marinade for a minimum of 3 hours.

Cooking your Air Fried Thai Haddock

1. Pre-heat your air fryer to 380°f.
2. Remove the haddock from the marinade and pour a little of the marinade into the baking tray, place the haddock in the baking tray and cook for 10 minutes turning midway.

Serving

Serve with salad.

Chicken Parmesan

Ingredients

4 Chicken Skinless Breasts

2 Eggs, lightly beaten

½ Cup Pork Rind Panko

¼ cup Almond Flour

½ Cup Parmesan Cheese, finely grated

1 tsp Italian Mixed Herbs

½ tsp Dried Garlic Powder

½ tsp Ground Black Pepper

¼ tsp Salt

Olive oil

Method

1. Mix together the pork rind panko, almond, parmesan, Italian mixed herbs, garlic powder, black pepper and salt in a large bowl.
2. Dip each of the chicken breasts in the beaten egg mix before tossing them into parmesan/herb mix, ensuring they are completely and evenly covered.

Cooking you Chicken Parmesan

1. Pre-heat your air fryer to 390°f.
2. Place the chicken breasts into the air fryer basket and cook for 10-12 minutes or until the chicken is golden.

Serving

Serve immediately, sliced, with salad.

3 Ingredient Battered Zucchini Bites

Ingredients

8-10 Zucchini Blossoms

1 Cup of Almond Flour

2 Eggs, lightly beaten

Salt and Ground Black Pepper to taste

Method

1. Mix the almond flour and a little salt and pepper in a mixing bowl.
2. Dip the zucchini blossoms into the egg mix, allowing any excess to drip back into the bowl.
3. Cover the zucchini in the almond flour mix and then straight into the air fryer.

Cooking your 4 Ingredients Battered Zucchini Bites

1. Pre-heat the air fryer to 380°f.
2. Add the zucchini to the air fryer basket and cook for 6-8 minutes or until the zucchini are crisp and golden in colour.

Serving

Serve hot alongside a yoghurt and lemon juice dip.

Dinner

High fat, moderate protein and low carb evening meals are essential to those currently in ketosis or those aiming to achieve it. The recipes featured in this section on the book really focus on real food that is easy to prepare, cost-effective and can be cooked up in little to no time at all. The meals have been tried and tested and have all proved to be delicious and in keeping with basic Ketogenic guidelines.

At the end of the chapter I had added a short section for snack items, some of which make the perfect Keto desert. Snacking on the Ketogenic diet can sometimes be tricky. I find that making my snacks in advance and storing them works great for me. It's the only sure-fire way to ensure that my snacks contain the amounts of specific ingredients that are required to get the best out of the Ketogenic diet and meal plan. Now, strictly speaking, ingredients like carrots aren't Keto, however, we will all need some low -level carbs from time to time and so I have included some snacks after the main course dishes, some of which contain low levels carbs, for example, Cinnamon Carrot sticks.

Coconut and Turmeric Chicken

Ingredients

4 Chicken quarters (whole leg pieces)

3tbl Coconut Paste

2tbl Turmeric

2 Inch piece of Ginger, grated

Salt and Ground Black Pepper to taste

Method

1. Combine coconut paste with all the spices in a mixing bowl.
2. Cut some deep slices into the chicken quarters. Evenly coat the chicken in the mix and leave to marinade for a minimum of 2 hours to overnight.

Cooking your Coconut and Turmeric Chicken

1. Pre-heat your air fryer to 380°f.
2. Cook the chicken pieces for 25 minutes (or until chicken is golden brown and any juices run clear, turn midway.

Serving

Serve hot.

Air Fried Cauliflower and Beef Hash

Ingredients

2 Fresh Chilies, finely sliced

2 Cloves of Garlic, grated

½ Onion, finely chopped

1 cup of Cauliflower, coarsely grated

400g Ground Beef

2 Eggs

Cooking your Air Fried Cauliflower and Beef Hash

1. Pre-heat your air fryer to 380°f.
2. Place the garlic, chilies, onion and ground beef into the air fryer's tray and cook for 8 minutes.
3. Pour away any excess fat and add the grated cauliflower to the ground beef and mix thoroughly. Place the tray back into the air fryer for 3-4 minutes.
4. Remove the tray from the air fryer and use a tablespoon to create 2 indentations in the mix, no deeper than 2 cm.
5. Crack the eggs, one into each indentation and carefully place the tray back into the air fryer and cook for a further 5 minutes.

Serving

Serve hot (3 servings).

Honey and Lime Chicken

Ingredients

4-6 Chicken Breasts

2 Cloves of Garlic finely chopped

¼tsp grated Ginger

2tbl Honey

2tbl freshly squeezed Lime Juice

1 Pinch of Chili Flakes

2tsp of Olive Oil

Salt and Ground Black Pepper to taste

Method

1. Combine the honey, olive oil, garlic, lime, chili flakes, salt, and ground black pepper to taste.
2. Cut some slices into the chicken breasts but, be careful don't cut all the way through. Place the chicken breasts in the honey and lime mix and leave to marinade for at least 2 hours to overnight.

Cooking you Honey and Lime Chicken

1. Pre-heat your air fryer to 360°f.

2. Place your honey and lime chicken breasts into the air fryer basket and cook for 20-25 minutes or until golden brown, turning midway.

Serving

Serve hot with rice or salad depending on your current carb intake.

Tandoori Chicken Quarters

Ingredients

2-4 Chicken Quarters

1½tsp Tandoori paste

1tsp Garlic Paste

1tsp Ginger Paste

½tbl Lemon Juice

Salt and Ground Black Pepper to taste

Method

1. Combine the tandoori paste, garlic paste, ginger paste, lemon juice and a little salt and ground black pepper to taste in a large mixing bowl.
2. Coat the chicken quarters in the tandoori paste mix and leave to marinade from a minimum of 2 hours to overnight.
3. Lightly spray the marinated chicken quarters with olive oil before cooking.

Cooking your Tandoori Chicken Quarters

1. Pre-heat your air fryer to 360°f.
2. Carefully place your tandoori chicken quarters in the air fryer basket and cook for 20-25

minutes or until golden brown and beginning to
crisp.

Serving

Serve with garlic seasoned potatoes or rice (optional).

Steak and Asparagus

Ingredients

Sirloin or Fillet Steaks

125g Asparagus

Olive Oil

Salt and Ground Black Pepper to taste

1tsp Butter

Method

1. Season the steaks with salt and ground black pepper and lightly spray with olive oil.
2. Season the asparagus with salt and ground black pepper and lightly spray with olive oil, put to one side.

Cooking your Air Fried Steak and Asparagus

1. Pre-heat your air fryer to 380°f for 5 minutes.
2. Place your Steaks onto the air fryer baking tray and cook for 6 minutes before turning and cooking for a further 3 minutes. When the Steaks have been cooking for 4 minutes, toss the Asparagus into the air fryer with the Steak.

Serving

Serve hot with salad and a little salt and butter for the asparagus.

Beer Batter Cod

Ingredients

2-4 Cod Fillets cleaned and de-shelled.

1 Cup Almond Flour

¼ tsp Baking Soda

½ tsp Paprika

1 tsp Salt

1 tsp Ground Black Pepper

½ Cup Beer of choice

Method

1. Start by mixing together the flour, baking soda, paprika, salt, pepper and beer in a bowl.
2. Whisk until the mixture is smooth.
3. Carefully dip the cod fillets in the beer batter, ensuring they are properly coated. Allow any excess batter to drip back into the mix.

Cooking your Beer Batter Cod

1. Line the bottom of your air fryer with foil and pre-heat your air fryer to 380°f.
2. Cook the beer batter cod for 10-12 minutes or until golden brown, turning midway

Serving

Serve hot with salad, salt, malt vinegar and squeeze of lemon.

Pan-Fried Seabass with Chili Butter

Ingredients

4-6 Sea bass fillets with the Skin still on.

100g Unsalted Butter

2 tbl Amarula Cream Liquor

1 Red Chili finely seeded and chopped

1 Green Chili, finely seeded and chopped

½ A Lime

Olive Oil

Salt and Ground Black Pepper

Method

1. Lightly whisk the butter, chilies, Amarula cream liquor, a squeeze of lime, and a little salt and pepper to taste.
2. Coat the seabass fillets with the mix and leave to marinate for at least 30 minutes.

Cooking your Pan-Fried Seabass with Chili Butter

1. Put the baking tray in the air fryer and pre-heat to 380°f.

2. Place the seabass skin down on to the baking tray and air fry for 3-5 minutes, hold the fish down with a spatula to stop it curling.
3. Turn and cook for a further 2 minutes.

Serving

Serve hot with salad or rice.

Sweet and Sticky Pork

Ingredients

4 Pork Loins

2 Cloves of Garlic finely chopped

1 Inch piece of Ginger, grated

1 tbl Honey

1 tbl Soy Sauce

¼ Ground Black Pepper

¼ tsp Mild Chili Powder

1 tsp Balsamic Vinegar

1 tbl Coconut Oil

Method

1. Mix all of the spices (half the ground black pepper), honey, coconut oil and soy sauce in a bowl.
2. Tenderise the pork loins, season with the ground pepper and cut them into strips.
3. Add the pork loin strips to the mix and fully cover.
4. Leave to marinade for a minimum of 2 hours up to overnight.

Cooking your Sweet and Sticky Pork

1. Pre-heat your air fryer to 380°f.
2. Place the pork loin strips along with the marinade into the baking tray and air fry/air bake for 8 minutes on each side or until golden brown.

Serving

Serve hot with fries (if your carbohydrate allowance allows it).

Keto Salmon Salad

Ingredients

1 Can of Salmon in Mineral Water, drained

1 Clove of Garlic, grated

½ Inch piece of fresh Ginger, grated

1 Pack of sun-Dried Tomatoes, chopped

1 tbl Lemon Juice

1 Cup of Romain Lettuce, roughly shredded

½ Cup of Spinach, roughly shredded

1 Spring Onion, chopped

Salt and Ground Black Pepper

Olive Oil

Method

1. Combine the salmon, ginger, garlic, sun-dried tomatoes, lemon juice, and a little salt and pepper to taste in a large mixing bowl.
2. Use your hands to form 3 patties from the mix, each being around 1 inch thick.
3. Lightly spray with olive oil before cooking.

Cooking your Keto Salmon Salad

3. Pre-heat your air fryer to 360°f.

4. Gently place the salmon patties into the air fryer basket and cook for 6-8 minutes.

Serving

Serve immediately atop a bed of lettuce, spring onion, and spinach.

Crab Stuffed Portobello Mushrooms

Ingredients

4 Portobello Mushrooms

110g Crab meat, finely chopped

4 Cloves of Garlic, grated

½ tsp Italian Mixed Herbs

½ cup Parmesan Cheese, grated

2 tbl Cream Cheese

½ tsp Paprika

Salt and Ground Black Pepper

1 tbl Parsley, chopped.

Olive Oil

Method

1. Cut the stems off the mushrooms, discard the stems and season the mushroom caps with a little salt and ground pepper to taste.
2. Mix the crab meat, garlic, Italian mixed herbs, cream cheese and paprika in a mixing bowl. Mix well.
3. Stuff the mushroom caps with the mix and generously sprinkle each stuffed mushroom with Parmesan cheese.
4. Lightly spray with olive oil before cooking.

Cooking your Crab Stuffed Portobello Mushrooms

1. Pre-heat your air fryer to 380°f.
2. Gently place the stuffed mushrooms into the air
    fryer basket and cook for 15 minutes or until
    the mushrooms are tender and the inner mix
    has a golden crust.

Serving

Top with chopped parsley and serve immediately.

Kimchi Pork Belly

Ingredients

300g Pork Belly

400g Kimchi

1 tbl Tamari

1 tbl rice wine

1 tsp Sesame seeds

1 Spring onion, finely chopped

Method

1. Thinly slice the pork belly and marinade in a mix of the tamari, rice wine for 30 minutes.
2. Cut the kimchi into 2cm pieces.
3. Lightly spray with olive oil before cooking.

Cooking your Kimchi Pork Belly

1. Pre-heat your air fryer to 380°f.
2. Place the marinated pork belly into the air fryer tray and cook for 10 minutes.
3. Add the kimchi to the tray and cook for a further 2-3 minutes.
4. Add the spring onion to the tray and cook for 1 minute further.

Serving

Serve hot.

Bombay Meatballs

Ingredients

450g ground Beef

2 Cloves of garlic, grated

1 Inch piece of Ginger, grated

½ Red Onion, finely chopped

1 tsp Cumin

1 ½ tsp Masala

¼ tsp Chilli Powder

Salt and Ground Black Pepper

Olive Oil

Method

1. Add the cooked onions, garlic and ginger (see below) to the ground beef, along with the masala, chili, cumin, and a little salt and ground black pepper to taste. Mix well.
2. Use your hands to roll meatball shapes from the ground beef mix and leave to sit for 5 minutes.
3. Lightly spray with olive oil before cooking.

Cooking your Bombay Meatballs

1. Pre-heat your air fryer to 360°f.
2. Place the onion, garlic, and ginger into the air fryer tray, spray once with olive oil and cook for

1-2 minutes. When cooked add to the ground beef.

3. Turn the air fryer up to 380°f.
4. Place the meatballs into the air fryer basket in batches of 4 and cook for 10-12 minutes or until the meatballs are golden and begin to crisp.

Serving

Serve hot.

Garlic Butter Scallops

Ingredients

8 Scallops

2 tbl Butter

2 Cloves of Garlic, grated

Ground Black Pepper

Olive Oil

Cooking your Garlic Butter Scallops

1. Pre-heat the air fryer to 360°f.
2. Add the grated garlic to the air fryer tray along with a light spray of oil and cook for 30 seconds.
3. Add the butter to the garlic and cook for a further 20 seconds.
4. Turn the air fryer up to 380°f.
5. Carefully place the Scallops into the butter and cook for 4 minutes, turning midway.

Serving

Serve immediately.

Scampi

Ingredients

6-8 Whole Scampi

3 tbl Butter

2 Cloves of garlic, grated

A pinch of Chili flakes

2 tbl White wine of choice

½ Fresh Lemon

Method

1. Place the butter, garlic, chili, into a saucepan and warm over a low heat for 2-3 minutes in order to melt the butter and infuse the ingredients.
2. Add the scampi to the butter sauce and stir well.

Cooking your Scampi

1. Pre-heat the air fryer to 330°f.
2. Pour the scampi and butter sauce into the air fryer pan and cook for 5 minutes.
3. Remove the pan and its contents from the air fryer and leave to sit for 1 minute.

Serving

Serve immediately with Avocado Fries.

Avocado Fries

Ingredients

1 Avocado

Salt and ground Black Pepper

Olive Oil

Method

1. Slice the Avocado in half and remove the stone.
2. cut each avocado half into 7 equal slices, carefully remove the skins and lightly season with salt and ground black pepper to taste.
3. Lightly spray with olive oil before cooking.

Cooking your Bacon Wrapped Asparagus

1. Pre-heat your air fryer to 360°f.
2. Toss the avocado into the air fryer basket and cook for 6-8 minutes or until the avocado is golden and beginning to crisp.

Serving

Serve immediately.

Tandoori Chicken Breast

Ingredients

2-4 Chicken Breasts

5 tbl yoghurt

½ Inch piece of fresh Ginger, grated

2 Cloves of Garlic, grated

1 tsp Chili powder

1 tsp Paprika

1 tsp Garam Masala

½ tsp Cayenne Pepper

½ tsp Salt

1 tsp Cumin

1 tsp Turmeric

Lemon Juice to garnish

Method

1. Mix the yoghurt, ginger, garlic, chili powder, paprika, garam masala, cayenne pepper, salt, cumin, turmeric in a large mixing bowl.
2. Cut the chicken breasts into strips and add to the marinade mix and leave to marinate for at least 30 minutes.

Cooking your Tandoori chicken breast

1. Pre-heat your air fryer to 380°f.
2. Gently place the marinated chicken breast strips into the air fryer basket and cook for 10-12 minutes or until the chicken begins to crisp.

Serving

Delicious both hot and cold with a squirt of lemon juice.

Coconut, Ginger and Turmeric Chicken

Ingredients

3-4 Chicken quarters (whole leg pieces)

3 tbl of Coconut Paste

2 tsp Turmeric

2 Inch piece of Ginger, grated

2 tsp Cayenne Pepper

¼ tsp Salt

½ tsp Ground Black Pepper

Method

1. Put the chicken to one side and mix all of the other ingredients together in a bowl.
2. Cut some deep slices into the chicken pieces and then fully coat the chicken in the mix and leave to marinade for a minimum of 2 hours to overnight.

Cooking your Coconut and Turmeric Chicken

1. Pre-heat your air fryer to 380°f.
2. Cook the chicken pieces for 20-22 minutes (or until chicken is golden and any juices run clear,

turn midway. Allow the coconut past marinade to crisp and darken at the edge this will enhance the overall flavour.

Serving

Serve hot.

Panko Fish sticks

Ingredients

450g Cod or other white fish of choice

½ Cup Panko Breadcrumbs

½ Cup Pork Rind Panko

1 tsp Cayenne Pepper

Salt and Ground Black Pepper

1 Egg, lightly beaten

Olive Oil

A squeeze of fresh lemon juice to garnish

Method

1. Mix together the panko breadcrumbs, pork rind panko, cayenne pepper, and a little salt and black pepper to taste. Be aware that the pork rind panko is itself rather salty and extra salt may not be required. Do a quick taste test on the mix before adding any salt to be safe.
2. Cut the cod into even parts around 6cm long and 2.5cm thick. Gently remove any excess moisture from the fish using kitchen towel.
3. Submerge each of the fish pieces in the egg mix and then toss into the panko mix ensuring they are completely and evenly covered.

Cooking your Panko Fish Sticks

1. Pre-heat your air fryer to 390°f.
2. Carefully place the fish sticks into the air fryer basket and cook for 8-10 minutes turning midway.

Serving

Serve hot, garnish with a squeeze of fresh lemon juice.

Crispy Pork Chops

Ingredients

4 boneless Porkchops

½ Cup Panko Breadcrumbs

2 tbl Almond Flour

1 tsp Turmeric

1 tsp paprika

½ tsp Ground Black Pepper

¼ tsp Salt

1 Egg, lightly beaten

Olive Oil

Method

1. Combine all the dry ingredients together in a large mixing bowl.
2. Submerge the pork chops one at a time on the egg mix and then put them into the panko mix ensuring that both sides of the pork chops are evenly covered.

Cooking your crispy Pork Chops

1. Pre-heat your air fryer to 400°f.
2. Place the pork chops in batches of two into the air fryer and cook for 12 minutes turning midway.

Serving

Serve hot.

Maple Mustard Chicken

Ingredients

4 Chicken Breasts

¼ Cup Mayonnaise

½ Cup Dijon Mustard

1 tsp English Mustard

¼ Cup low-sugar Maple Syrup

Salt and Ground Black Pepper

Method

1. Mix the mayonnaise, Dijon and English mustard, maple syrup, and a little salt and ground black pepper to taste.
2. Cut each chicken breast into 4-5 slices and submerge them in the maple marinade mix and leave to rest for at least two hours but preferably overnight.

Cooking you Maple Mustard Chicken

1. Pre-heat your air fryer to 380°f.
2. Place the marinated chicken breast strips into the air fryer basket and cook for 10-12 minutes turning midway.

Serving

Serve hot with avocado fires or air fried garlic sprouts.

Oriental Chicken and broccoli

Ingredients

2 Chicken Breast

3 Cups Broccoli

3 Cloves of garlic, grated

1 Inch piece of Ginger, grated

3 Spring Onions, finely chopped

3 tbl Soy Sauce

2 tsp Fish Sauce

1 tsp Sesame Oil

Method

1. Cut the chicken breasts into strips and put to one side.
2. Warm a saucepan over a medium heat and add the garlic along with a little olive oil.
3. Add the ginger, spring onions, soy sauce, fish sauce, and sesame oil to the pan along with the chicken strips and cook for 5 minutes.
4. Spoon 2-3 tbl of the marinade over the broccoli florets and put them to one side.

Cooking you Oriental Chicken and Broccoli

1. Pre-heat your air fryer to 380°f.

2. Carefully place the chicken and into the air fryer tray with 2 tbl of the marinade mix and cook for 5 minutes.

3. Remove the tray from the air fryer and place the chicken and broccoli into the air fryer basket and cook for 8 minutes or until the broccoli begins to crisp.

Serving

Serve immediately.

Soy Sauce and Apple Cod with Fennel and Dill

Ingredients

2 Cod Fillets

2 Clove of Garlic, grated

½ Piece of Fresh Ginger, grated

1 tsp Ground Fennel Seeds

1 tsp Dried Dill

3 tbl Soy Sauce

2 tbl Sesame Oil

Salt and Ground Black Pepper to taste

6 Sprigs of Fresh Dill, finely chopped

1 Fennel Bulb, finely sliced

1 Apple, sliced.

Method

1. Mix the garlic, ground Fennel Seeds, ginger, dried dill, Soy Sauce, and 1 tbl of sesame oil.
2. Season the cod with salt and ground black pepper and place the cod in the marinade for a minimum of 30 minutes up to 3 hours or as long as overnight.

Garnish

1. In a separate bowl mix the sliced apple, fennel,
    dill, 1 tbl of sesame oil and a little salt and
    ground black pepper to taste.

**Cooking your Soy Sauce and Apple Cod with
Fennel and Dill**

1. Put the baking tray into your air fryer and pre-
    heat your air fryer to 380°f.
2. Place the marinate cod fillets in the air fryer and
    cook for 8 minutes or until they are golden
    brown.

Serving

Serve hot with the sliced apple, fennel and dill garnish.

Air Fried Keto Sausage Bites

Ingredients

450g Seasoned Pork/Italian Sausage

1 Cup Cheddar Cheese, grated

½ Cup Almond Flour

1 Egg

1 tsp Cayenne Pepper

1 tsp Dried Garlic Powder

1 tsp Dried Onion Powder

Olive Oil

Method

1. Combine all of the ingredients in a large mixing bowl.
2. Using your hands form 12-14 equal sized balls from the mix.
3. Lightly spray with olive oil before cooking.

Cooking your Air Fired Keto Sausage Bites

1. pre-heat your air fryer to 400°f.
2. Place the sausage balls into the air fryer in batches of 4 and cook for 10 minutes or until the sausage bites begin to crisp.

Serving

Serve immediately.

Crab Cakes

Ingredients

400g Fresh or Tinned Crabmeat

¼ Cup Almond Flour

1 tsp Ground Black Pepper

¼ tsp Dried Garlic Powder

¼ tsp Dried Ginger Powder

Olive Oil

Method

1. Combine the crabmeat, almond, ground black pepper, garlic and ginger in a large bowl.
2. Use your hands to form patty shapes from the crabmeat mix.
3. Lightly spray from olive oil before cooking.

Cooking your Crab Cakes

1. pre-heat your air fryer to 380°f.
2. Place the crab cakes into the air fryer basket for 8-10 minutes (turning midway) or until the crab cakes turn golden.

Serving

Serve Immediately.

Air Fried Crispy Chicken Thighs

Ingredients

4-6 Large Chicken thighs

3 Cloves of Garlic, grated

½ Piece of Ginger, grated

2 tbl Olive Oil

Salt and Ground Black Pepper

Method

1. Mix the garlic, ginger, and olive oil in a mixing bowl along with a little salt and pepper to taste.
2. Add the chicken thighs to the bowl and stir, ensuring they are all fully coated with the olive oil and garlic mix.

Cooking you Air Fried Crispy Chicken Thighs

1. pre-heat your air fryer to 400°f.
2. Place the chicken thighs into the air fryer basket and cook for 10-12 minutes or until the chicken is crispy and golden in colour.

Serving

Serve hot.

Lamb Koftas

Ingredients

450g Ground Lamb

3 Cloves of Garlic, grated

½ White Onion, finely chopped

1 tsp Oregano

1 tsp Cayenne Pepper

1 tsp Ground Black Pepper

¼ tsp Salt

Olive Oil

Skewers- wooden or metal

Method

1. If you are using wooden skewers it is important that you soak them in cold water for at least half an hour prior to cooking to stop them from burning in the air fryer.
2. Mix the ground lamb, garlic, onion, oregano, cayenne pepper, black pepper, and salt in a mixing bowl.
3. Use your hands to form sausage shapes from the ground lamb and seasoning mix and push a skewer vertically through each of the koftas.
4. Lightly spray with olive oil before cooking.

Cooking you Lamb Koftas

1. Pre-heat your air fryer to 400°f.
2. Cook the lamb koftas for 10-12 minutes or until golden.

Serving

Serve hot with a cool dipping sauce.

Garlic Fried Mushrooms

Ingredients

2 Cups Creminis or Button Mushrooms, halved

2 eggs, lightly beaten

¼ Cup Almond Flour

¼ Cup Pork Rind Panko

2 tsp of Garlic Powder

1 tsp Mixed Herbs

1 tsp Ground Black Pepper

¼ tsp Salt

Method

1. Mix the garlic, mixed herbs, almond flour, panko, salt and ground black pepper in a mixing bowl.
2. Dip each of the mushrooms into the beaten egg mix, allow any excess to drip back into the bowl and then place them into the flour and herb mix.
3. Ensure all the mushrooms are fully covered in the mix.

Cooking your Garlic Fried Mushrooms

1. Pre-heat the air fryer to 380°f.
2. Place the mushrooms into the air fryer tray and cook for 10-12 minutes or until golden.

Serving

Serve hot as the perfect appetiser.

Snacks

Brussel Sprout Chips

Ingredients

2 Cups of Brussel Sprouts

Salt and Ground Black Pepper

Method

1. Thinly slice the Brussel sprouts using a sharp knife.
2. Season the Brussel sprouts with salt and ground black pepper and lightly spray with oil.

Cooking you Brussel Sprout Chips

1. Pre-heat the air fryer to 360°f.
2. Place the Brussel sprouts into the air fryer basket and cook for 8-9 minutes.

Serving

Serve immediately.

Kale Crisps

Ingredients

2 cups Kale

1tbl Olive Oil

Salt to taste

1tsp Soy Sauce

Method

1. Wash and dry the kale.
2. Remove the stems and tear the kale into 2-inch pieces.
3. Mix the kale with the soy sauce and olive oil and add a little salt.

Cooking your Kale Crisps

1. Pre-heat your air fryer to 200°f.
2. Put the kale into the air fryer and cook for 3 minutes, tossing halfway through.

Serving

Serve hot or cold with extra salt if required.

Asian Style Cucumber Crisps

Ingredients

1 Whole Cucumber

2 Cloves of Garlic, grated

1tbl Soy Sauce

¼ Cup of Flour

1tsp Paprika

2tsp Cayenne Pepper

1tsp Sugar

Salt and Ground Pepper to taste

1tbl Olive Oil

Method

1. Mix the soy sauce, olive oil, garlic, sugar, salt and pepper in a bowl.
2. In a separate bowl mix the flour, cayenne pepper, paprika and a little salt and ground pepper to taste.
3. Add the Cucumber slices into the soy sauce mix and stir. Leave to marinade for at 10 minutes.

4. Remove the cucumber from the soy sauce and throw them into the flour mix, making sure they are fully coated. Shake off any excess flour.
5. Lightly spray with olive oil before cooking.

Cooking your Asian Style Cucumber Crisps

1. Pre-heat your air fryer to 360°f.
2. Place the cucumber slices in the air fryer basket in a haphazard fashion and cook for around 3 minutes or until crisp. Turn midway.

Serving

Serve hot or cold with a sprinkling of salt/sugar mix.

Crispy Seaweed

Ingredients

2 cups Kale destemmed Kale Leaves

1 tsp Shrimp Powder (available at Asian supermarkets)

¼ tsp Sugar

¼ tsp Salt

1 tbl Sesame Seeds

Method

1. Put the kale leaves together and roll them up into a tight cylinder.
2. Finely slice the kale into thin strips.
3. Boil a saucepan of water on a medium heat. Toss the kale strips into the water and blanch (boil) for 30 seconds.
4. Remove the kale strips from the water and dry with kitchen towel.
5. Sprinkle with salt, sugar and shrimp powder.

Cooking your Crispy Seaweed

1. Pre-heat your air fryer to 360°f.
2. Toss the crispy seaweed into the air fryer basket and cook for 1 minute, tossing midway.

Serving

Delicious hot or cold.

Air Fried Blueberry Muffins

Ingredients

½ Cup of Almond Flour

2 tbl Coconut Flour

2 Eggs

1 tsp Cinnamon

1 tsp Baking Soda

1 tsp Vanilla Extract

½ Cup Coconut Oil

¼ Cup Almond Milk

¼ Cup Raspberries

½ Cup Blueberries

Olive Oil

Method

1. Mix together the almond and coconut flour along with the cinnamon and baking soda in a large mixing bowl.
2. Add the eggs, vanilla extract, coconut oil and almond milk to the flours/cinnamon mix and mix until combined.

3. Toss the raspberries and blueberries into the mix and stir well.
4. Use your hands to create 4-6 patties from the dough around 3cm/1 inch thick.
5. Lightly spray with olive oil before cooking.

Cooking your Air Fried Blueberry Muffins

1. Pre-heat your air fryer to 350°f.
2. Place the blueberry muffins into the air fryer basket in batches of 3 at a time and cook for 14-26 minutes or until golden.

Serving

Allow to cool before serving.

Air Fried Salami-Wrapped Mozzarella

Ingredients

Mozzarella sticks

Salami

Red Onion Relish

Olive Oil

Toothpicks

Method

1. Chop the mozzarella sticks into quarters.
2. Wrap each of the mozzarella quarters with salami and pin in place using a toothpick.

Cooking your Air Fried Salami Wrapped Mozzarella

1. Pre-heat your air fryer to 350°f.
2. Place the salami wrapped mozzarella pieces into the air fryer basket and cook for 5 minutes.

Serving

Serve immediately with a red onion relish for the perfect snack or appetiser.

Garlic Sprouts

Ingredients

2 Cups of Brussel Sprouts

3 Cloves of Garlic, grated

Olive Oil

Method

1. Mix the grated garlic with 2 tbl olive oil in a large bowl. Stir well and leave to sit for at least ten minutes.
2. Add the Brussel sprouts to the mixing bowl and stir well ensuring that all the sprouts are evenly coated in the olive oil and garlic mix.

Cooking your Garlic Sprouts

1. Pre-heat your air fryer to 360°f.
2. Place the garlic sprouts into the air fryer basket and cook for 8-10 minutes, or until the sprouts are crisp on the outside and tender inside.

Serving

Serve immediately.

Garlic Fried Broccoli

Ingredients

2 Cups of Organic Broccoli, chopped into florets

3 Cloves of Garlic, grated

Olive Oil

Method

1. Mix the grated garlic with 2 tbl olive oil in a large bowl. Stir well and leave to sit for at least ten minutes.
2. Add the broccoli to the mixing bowl and stir well ensuring that all the florets are evenly coated in the olive oil and garlic mix.

Cooking your Garlic Fried Broccoli

1. Pre-heat your air fryer to 360°f.
2. Place the broccoli into the air fryer basket and cook for 8-10 minutes, or until the broccoli begins to crisp.

Serving

Serve immediately.

Cinnamon Carrot Sticks

Ingredients

2 Carrots

2 tsp Cinnamon

1 tsp Turmeric

Salt and Ground Black Pepper

Olive Oil

Method

1. Wash the carrots (leave the skin on) and cut them into stick around 5cm long and 1½cm thick.
2. Coat the carrot sticks with a generous sprinkling of cinnamon and turmeric followed by a little salt and ground black pepper.

Cooking your Cinnamon Carrot Sticks

1. Pre-heat your air fryer to 380°f.
2. Toss the carrot sticks into the air fryer basket and cook for 10-12 minutes, shake up the air fryer basket midway.

Serving

Serve hot.

Cayenne Crabsticks

Ingredients

1 Packet of Crabsticks

1 Cayenne Pepper

¼ tsp Paprika

½ tsp Turmeric

2 tsp Olive Oil

Method

1. Mix the olive oil, cayenne pepper, paprika, and turmeric in a bowl.
2. Place the crabsticks into the olive oil and cayenne mix and make sure they are fully coated. Let any excess mix drip back into the bowl.

Cooking your Cayenne Crabsticks

1. Pre-heat your air fryer to 340°f.
2. Air fry your Crabsticks for 10 minutes tossing regularly to ensure they are cooking evenly.

Serving

Serve hot or cold.

Air Roasted Spicy Chickpeas

Ingredients

1 Tin of Chickpeas, drained

1 tbl Olive Oil

1 tsp Mixed Spice

1 tsp Cayenne Pepper

¼ tsp Salt

Method

1. Pat dry your chickpeas with some kitchen towel and toss them into a bowl along with your mixed spice, cayenne pepper, salt, and olive oil and mix well to make sure all of the chickpeas are coated in the olive oil mix.

Cooking your Air Roasted Spicy Chickpeas

2. Pre-heat your air fryer to 390°f.
3. Cook the Chickpeas at 390°f for 8-10 minutes tossing regularly.

Serving

Serve warm in a bowl as a delicious starter or table snack.

Air Fried Artichoke Hearts

Ingredients

6 Artichoke Hearts cut into halves

1 Cup of Almond Flour

½ tsp Salt

1 tsp Ground Black Pepper

Method

1. Mix the almond flour, salt, and pepper in a bowl.
2. Add the artichokes to the bowl and mix, ensuring they are evenly covered in the almond flour mix.
3. Lightly spray with olive oil before cooking.

Cooking your Fried Artichoke Hearts

1. Pre-heat your air fryer to 380°f.
2. Air fry the artichoke hearts for 4-5 minutes or until golden brown, tossing regularly.

Serving

Serve hot with tartar sauce.

Air Fried Spicy Battered Okra

Ingredients

400g Okra

½ Cup Almond Flour

2 Eggs, lightly beaten

½ tsp Paprika

1 tsp Turmeric

½ tsp Cayenne Pepper

½ tsp Medium Heat Chilli Powder

½ tsp Salt

Method

1. Combine the flour, cayenne pepper, salt and paprika in a bowl.
2. Chop the okra into cubes.
3. Dip and fully submerge the okra pieces in the beaten egg mix, allowing any excess to drip back into the bowl.
4. Coat the okra in the almond flour and spice mix.

Cooking your Battered Okra

1. Pre-heat your air fryer to 380°f.
2. Cook the battered okra for 4-5 minutes or until golden brown.

Serving

Serve hot.

Air Fried Coconut Chai Snack Bars

Ingredients

½ Cup Chia Seeds

½ Cup Cashew nuts

1 Cup dried Coconut flesh, shredded or roughly grated

½ Cup fresh water

1 tbl Coconut oil

1 tbl Honey

¼ tsp Vanilla Extract

1 tsp cinnamon

Method

1. Soak the chia seeds in the ½ cup of fresh water for 12-15 minutes or until they soften.
2. Remove the chia seeds form the water and allow any excess water to drip away before putting the chai in a large mixing bowl.
3. Add the coconut, cashews, coconut oil, vanilla extract, honey, and cinnamon to the bowl and mix until the ingredients are fully combined.
4. Use your hands to form 6-8 rectangle shapes around 2cm thick.

Cooking your Air Fried Coconut Chai Snack Bars

1. Pre-heat the air fryer to 360°f.
2. Place the coconut chai bars into the air fryer tray and cook for 20-22 minutes or until the edges are crisp, turn regularly.

Serving

Allow to cool before eating.

Air fried Hazelnut Cookies

Ingredients

2 Cups Hazelnuts

60g Butter

2 Eggs

½ Almond Flour

¼ cup Tapioca Flour

½ Cup Coconut Sugar

¼ tsp Vanilla Extract

A pinch of Salt

Method

1. Toss the hazelnuts into a food processor and pulse until the nuts have been processed to a consistency like a coarse flour.
2. Add the rest of the ingredients together and blend until they begin to form a dough like texture.
3. Use your hands to form small balls from the dough, then using your palm gently squash the dough into cookie shapes around 1cm thick.

Cooking your Air Fried Hazelnut Cookies

1. Pre-heat the air fryer to 360°f.

2. Place the cookies in batches of four into the air fryer basket and cook for 12 minutes, turning midway.

Serving

Allow to cool.

Pineapple Fritters

Ingredients

1 Pack/tin of Pineapple Rings

1 Cup of Almond Flour

2 Eggs

¼ Cup Milk

2 Tbl Coconut sugar

Method

1. In a bowl whisk the almond flour, eggs, milk, and coconut sugar until smooth.
2. Generously coat the pineapple rings in the batter mix.

Cooking you Pineapple Fritter

1. Pre-heat your air fryer to 380°f.
2. Line the air fryer basket with foil and cook the pineapple fritters for 3 minutes or until golden brown. Turn midway.

Serving

Serve hot with a sprinkling of cinnamon and/or ice cream.